OVERCOMING DEPRESSION

OVERCOMING DEPRESSION

By Claudie Marielle Camann
& Dennis Toro Toro

Your Claudie & Dennis in summer 2020

:

Foreword for the Second Edition

Hi, my name is Dennis. It's great that you took the time to read our brief introduction. When it comes to guides and books, I am always interested in who wrote them and why. Therefore, I'd like to share the following statement with you: This book, in its second edition, (the first one was German) is a work of passion with the desire to inform. It's all about depression. Claudie and I share a passion for the human psyche and the soul. The time up to this moment in which you read these lines was an exciting one and characterized by a lively exchange. However, as all human things tend to be imperfect, this book might contain something that you find imperfect.

Please do share your feedback—it will be greatly appreciated. You can find our contact details at the end of the book.

I hope you enjoy reading it.

Table of Contents

Foreword for the Second Edition............5

Introduction 2

Depression - An Introduction 6

What is depression? 9

Outdated definition 9

The current definition of depression 10

What happens with depression? 11

Who is at risk? 13

Depression in facts and figures.............13

Recognize Depression.............18

Causes.............19

The genes.............23

Environmental influences.............25

Stressors 26

Psycho-trauma.............28

Biochemical changes 30

Resilience.............30

Sleep disorder.............31

Pregnancy 33

Symptoms.............34

But what are the differences? 34

Depression in Children 36

The Diversity of Depression.............41

Differential diagnostics.............41

Dysthymia 42

Seasonal affective disorder.............42

Bipolar disorder 44

Schizoaffective disorder.............45

Depressed mood 46

Depressive episode.............46

Recurrent depressive disorder............................47
Adjustment disorder................................48
Chronic depression 48
Depression and other mental illnesses.................49
A far-reaching disease 51
The Meaning of Depression 53
For the affected 54
For the environment................................56
For the job 57
Understanding.....................................60
Not a broken leg yet still restricted 64
For Relatives 65
How should I make guesses? 66
What you can do to deal with the disease 68
Ten ideas for dealing with those affected 69
Self-help groups for relatives.........................74
A Way Out of Depression...........................75
Therapeutic approaches..............................76
Medical therapy....................................77
Psychotherapy 79
Behavioral therapy 80
Psychotherapy based on depth psychology.............81
Humanistic Psychotherapy9 82
Support groups 84
Relaxation techniques 86
What other therapy options are there?.................87
Goals of therapy for depression 92
What can I do?....................................93
What can I do if I have depression myself? 93
What can I do for a depressed person?.................99
This is how you can tell if therapy is working 102
Chances of recovery...............................105

Statistics and Figures 107
Author Note: In the End is the Beginning 109

Introduction
by C. Marielle Camann

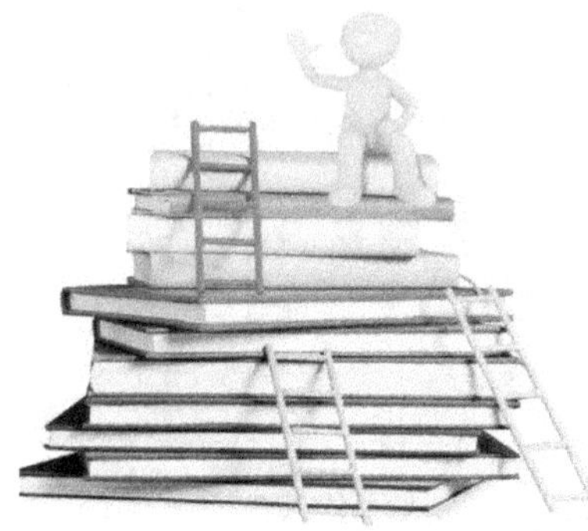

Dear readers,
I would like to welcome you to t his book. The presented topics portant to all of us!
Hardly any other disease is as drastic for the soul as are mental illnesses

Depression can have many different manifestations. Depression can often occur together with other mental illnesses, such as anxiety disorders or panic disorders. But even on its own, depression is a disease that can bring a lot of suffering. The suffering is felt not only by those affected by it but also by their relatives and loved ones.

The symptoms can often lead to an entirely wrong diagnosis and, in this way, fuel a vicious cycle that is extremely difficult to break. Frustration on both sides, discouragement, and a lot of pain: depression drains everything out of your body. However, depression can be treated and the chances of recovery are excellent. This is especially true if It is diagnosed early. People who are depressed rarely go to their doctor at the first sign and relatives also find it hard to classify the psychological changes at first. One can only assume at this stage as the changes could be due to a myriad reason.

Depression has many faces and expresses itself uniquely. If you are not a professional, it is difficult to recognize the first warning signs. Depression does not develop instantly. In most cases, it is a gradual process!

This also applies to burnout – a condition the depressed eventually suffer from. Nobody wakes up the next morning with a fully developed mental illness like depression or burnout. As such, it is not feasible to accurately identify too early and to understand the frequent malaise properly.

It is not uncommon for it to take weeks or even months to diagnose depression. It has such a complex appearance because it intervenes in so many bodily processes that it can hide behind unclear abdominal pain or headaches. However, once the diagnosis of depression has been made, many questions arise. What are the causes? How could it have advanced so far? But above all: how does it go on now?

Another problem is that many symptoms cannot be traced back to depression alone but often point to burnout as well. This makes the diagnosis even more complicated, as depression and burnout have a lot in common. Fear and existing panic attacks can also not be assigned to one of the two diseases. Varied effects on the body and mind make the diagnosis more intrinsic. This requires a certain amount of patience and extensive observation of the symptoms.

The affected and their relatives are presented with a fait accompli; feeling like they're at doctors' mercy, and yet have so many queries. The purpose of this book is to help solve that.

It should not only explain how depression expresses itself, but also what depression is. Recognizing depression is especially important to act quickly. In addition to the causes, I would also like to present the symptoms to you simultaneously. Moreover, you will find a personal check at the end of the book to see whether you or a loved one might be suffering from depression.

We already mentioned the versatility of the disease-- and it is! -- how it differs from other diseases like burnout and what forms it takes will also be part of this book. But depression is not only diverse but it is also far-reaching. It intervenes in many living spaces, challenges the sick person's social environment, and often donates displeasure and impatience. Those suffering and their families can quickly become overwhelmed and helpless in day-to-day activities. It need not be the case, though! There are ways out of depression as well as out of burnout! The relatives should also not be forgotten since they too can suffer enormously from the disease, and therefore will
discuss their case later on.
Relationships of all kinds are severely tested and pushed to by depression or burnout. Consequently, not only those affected need support, but also their immediate relatives and friends. Assistance, understanding, and measures that lead to the improved current situation can already bring about a major change here. Unfortunately, the relatives are all too often forgotten when looking at depression or burnout and further treatment.
Depression is a difficult disorder to understand. Those affected

do not have a bruise, do not hobble, and do not wear a cast around their feet: it is an invisible disease that needs salient treatment. But with more understanding of the relatives and better communication with those affected, plenty could be achieved.

Burnout is the same in its complexity and underlying behavior. The profound state of exhaustion often encounters resentment or a strong lack of understanding among outsiders, as the person's problems are challenging to understand.
We want to invite you now to take a trip into the world of depression. Please get to know the disease with us and find out what depression is all about.

Also, learn what the difference between depression and burnout is. With the increasing spread of depression and burnout, it is even more critical today to recognize its characteristics and similarities.

Depression - An Introduction

Depression is a serious mental illness. Whenever the soul calls for help, action needs to be taken. Depression is such a diverse and complex disorder that it is not always easy to identify. The most common association with depression is a lowering of mood or feeling "sad". A loss of interest in previously enjoyable hobbies and activities and a lack of drive or motivation are considered as the common symptoms. Depression consists of significantly more symptoms: irregular sleep cycle, being unable to sleep properly at night, self-doubt, ideas of worthlessness, and a lack of concentration.

The suicide rate of depressed people is 10 -15 percent! So, depression is more than just a sunken mood.

But unlike a broken leg, depression cannot be fathomed from the outside until it can no longer be hidden. The suffering of people with depression tends to go on for a long time. We are talking about a period of years in which depression can develop at an exponential pace.

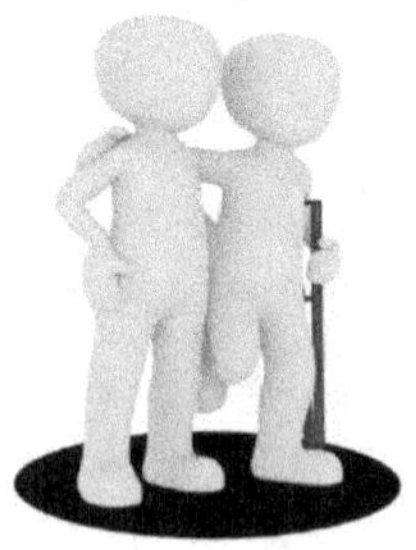

Depression can have a diverse appearance. Although there are clearly defined criteria, depression always expresses itself a little uniquely in each person. Some people would consider depression as an octopus that pulls one into a deep black hole with its powerful arms. Others might draw a comparison to a weaker self who keeps those affected by depression on a tight leash. Between exultant and emotionally petrified - depression offers a wide range of symptoms. A person affected must first be able to assess this and learn how to deal with it. By the time those affected notice what is happening, the depression has the patient firmly in its grasp.

This chapter is intended to give you an introductory overview of this widespread mental illness. Every year. 2 out of 100[1] people in Germany develop this mental illness. But what is depression, and what goes on in the brain of a person affected by it? These and other questions will be answered within this chapter.

[1] www.neurologen-und-psychiater-im-netz.org access 08-20

What is depression?

With the advancement of science in mental illnesses and research, depression research has flourished as well Over time, the definition of depression has changed. Most of the time, the outdated clinical definition can still be found in many people's hearts and minds. This circumstance often leads to a problem. Therefore, we would like to discuss the outdated and latest definition of depression.

Outdated definition

It was only a few years ago that the definition of the disease was divided into endogenous and exogenous depression. It was less about the symptoms than about the causes. Endogenous depression postulated that the disease started without a visible or organic trigger. It was usually assumed that there was a metabolic disorder in the brain, to which the genes were often ascribed as the primary cause. On the other hand, there was the exogenous depression, which required having a direct trigger: an organic disease or trauma.

Today this definition is seen as outdated and therefore is no longer applicable. One of the primary reasons is that medicine has made significant progress in depression research.

The current definition of depression

Depression is divided into three different degrees of severity: mild, moderate, and severe. However, it becomes more confusing with a clear differentiation between depressed mood, depressive episode, recurrent depressive disorder, adjustment disorder, chronic depression, or bipolar disorder. We will deal with all these different forms in more detail in the chapter "The Diversity of The Disease".

How is the onset of depression described according to the current definition (as of 2021 according to ICD 10)?

The onset of depression is said to begin as soon as two of the three main symptoms (lowering mood, reduction of energy, and decrease in activity) have existed continuously for 2 or more weeks.
Since the three main symptoms are common moods, they are not enough to identify depression even in healthy people. Here the seven so-called additional symptoms are consulted, of which at least two must persist over the same period. The seven additional symptoms of depression are:
- Difficulty concentrating and paying attention
- Dwindling and lack of self-esteem
- Self-doubt
- Feelings of guilt,
- Feelings of worthlessness
- Negative and grim prospects for the future
- Suicidal tendencies and intentions
- Sleep problems, difficulty falling asleep and staying

asleep.

- Weight loss or weight gain.

The more pronounced the more symptoms apply, the more likely it is to have moderate or severe depression. So nowadays, the diagnosis is based on this assessment.

What happens with depression?

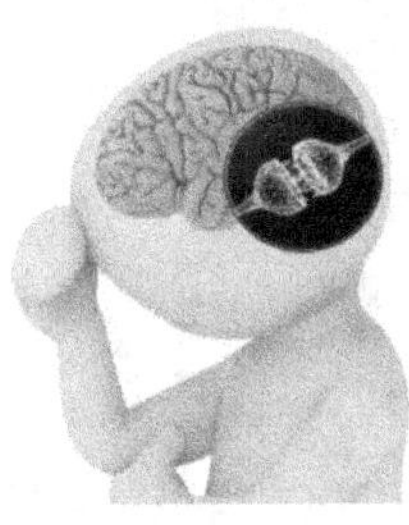

This is where it gets fascinating. Depression does not only necessarily require physical causes, but it is also an organic disease.

To understand what goes on in depression, you have to look into the human brain because it is the psyche in control and the origin of this disease. To do this, we zoom in very close and see that we are at the synapses. Synapses transmit and process the stimuli in the brain using so-called messenger substances. In depression, the messenger substances that act as a ferry between synapses are out of balance. Imagine that you are standing with a lot of people at an investor. The jetty is a synapse, and you want to reach the opposite bank with the other people to another synapse.

You and the people waiting with you at the jetty are the brain processes or stimuli. For example, you want to visit your parents while other people may want to tell them that the weather is nice today or something similar. Now everyone is waiting for the ferry. This comes too. Shortly before the jetty, she breaks and drives back onto the river. Ferries often run between the landing stages, but now it takes a long time.

Meanwhile, real crowds are piling up at the pier, all waiting for a ferry that doesn't come. Then finally there is a ferry again, but it can only take 3 people. Chaos arises, and the messages that people want to convey are not passed on due to the disrupted ferry service. And to put it very simply, that's exactly what happens when you're depressed.

Nerve stimuli are not or only sparsely transported due to the imbalance of the messenger substances. Can't these messenger substances simply be replenished? Unfortunately, no! It's not that simple. The drugs used today against depression have exactly this task, but this process involves interactions.

So, it's not all simple to fix this problem. But since the human brain is changeable, can build new structures, and create new nerve connections, new plexuses can be created in the brain. That is why psychotherapy, in addition to the well-renowned drug therapy, is of the greatest importance!

Who is at risk?

No one is immune from falling to depression. Still, there are people who are more likely to develop depression based on various factors. People who consume drugs or alcohol large amounts are more likely to develop depression than people addicted to drugs or alcohol. Of course, genes also play an important role. If you have already suffered from depression in your family, you belong to the risk group.

Older people who spend a lot of time alone - with little or no social contact - also belong to the risk group. The same applies to young people. Additionally, they have social and psychological stress that can also lead to depression. Similarly, there Is also an increased risk of developing depression for those who have already suffered from depression.

A thyroid dysfunction, for example, also leads to depression. It is now estimated that around 20-25% of women and 7-12% of men develop depression[2]. However, the actual number of cases is likely to be higher due to under-reporting of cases. While we're with the numbers, we would like to present the depression in facts and figures for support.

Depression in facts and figures

It is no longer a secret that depression is a serious illness. Yet, it is often not noticed, or accepted.
speak their own, sometimes frightening,

language. on this, illustrating the suffering and the seriousness of depression:

The North Rhine-Westphalia Chamber of Psychotherapists has published many facts and figures

Approximately 5 million people in Germany, or 8.3% of the population, suffer from depression[3]. However, the risk of developing depression at least once in a lifetime is significantly higher. For example, Europe and the USA the rate is 16 to 20% which is much higher.

For someone who is diagnosed and does not seek treatment, a depressive episode lasts about six to eight months, with half of the sick people having to go through another episode of depression soon. The risk of relapse increases to 70% after the second episode (4). Those who suffered from depression for the third time have a relapse risk of over 90 %. Interestingly enough, depression goes up to 60% associated with other mental illnesses such as addiction, anxiety disorders, cardiovascular diseases, migraines or diabetes mellitus. The list of possible diseases is very long.

---

[2] Depressive illnesses [Health Reporting - Special Issues, September 2010], http: //www.gbe-bund.de Access 08-20

3 https://www.ptk-nrw.de/de/lösungen/publikationen/ptk-newsletter/archiv/ptk-newsletter-special / numbers-facts-depression.html Access 08-20

Most people with depression see their GP sooner or later. The problem with this is that around 53% of all people suffering from depression do not get beyond the family doctor's treatment. Only 7% of those affected received psychotherapeutic help, while 4% were able to benefit from a combination of treatment from their family doctor and benefit from psychotherapy. What is the reason for this low percentage? The problem lies in the diagnosis. The more pronounced and severe the depression, the more likely it can be diagnosed. In 80% of cases, depression is only diagnosed in the severe depression stage!

A look at the suicide rate reveals how serious the disease is. Every twelfth patient tends to attempt suicide and fails or dies as a result of it! This is an enormous rate.

---

2 https://www.ptk-nrw.de/de/lösungen/publikationen/ptk-newsletter/archiv/

Recognize Depression

Detecting depression at an early stage and significantly increasing the chances of recovery is what matters. Now you have learned about the risk groups and those who are more likely to develop depression. These people should pay close attention to their mood and condition! People from the risk group can get it "ice cold."

Depression arises in the brain due to an imbalance in the messenger substances that transmit the stimuli. So, it's no wonder that this imbalance can affect just about anyone. In order to recognize it early, you should know its causes.

Of course, if you want to recognize depression, it is good to know what causes it. But the causes alone do not make depression so that we will look at the symptoms of depression. The connection between cause and symptoms is particularly important when identifying depression! This chapter also has many interesting and worth knowing facts ready for you.

Indeed, you are powerless against the genes, and nevertheless, we would like to send you some good news at this point:
No gene can be held responsible for the outbreak of depression!

How the individual causes lead to the fact that a person can suffer from depression is the aim of this chapter.

We also take a closer look at resilience (mental resistance) and sleep disorders. Pregnant women belong to this risk group of suffering from depression.

Causes

Research into the causes is of great importance. The causes for those affected are not always clear at first glance but before we delve into this topic, let's start at the very beginning.

There may be times that the depression has a cause; A distinction is made between two aspects: All causes can be divided between these two categories. However, you should, at this point push stereotypical thinking aside.
It is not the case here that there is only one cause! There are usually several causes that need to be treated together. There is an interaction between the two aspects. Depression is not purely physical (neurobiological) or purely psychosocial, but both sides must always be examined and treated!

Note: Depression is a mental illness, but it also clearly has a physical part. Please think of the ferry traffic from the previous chapter. There is no pure breakdown or classification, based on the motto: "Either, or "!

	Psychosocial	Neurobiological
Increased susceptibili ty	For example, triggered by a trauma or a traumatic experience.	For example, through the genes; this is where inheritance comes in.
Trigger	Negative or positive. For example, through the death of a loved one; stress, but also a wedding or a vacation trip.	For example, a dysfunction in the stress hormone balance: adrenaline, noradrenaline, and cortisol are released continuously and cortisol is released when needed.

Status	Often, joylessness and hopelessness.	Here, for example, an imbalance can be demonstrated, which affects the messenger substance regions of the brain
Therapy	Psychotherapy	Therapy based on drugs.

Age is also interesting. It is questionable whether this can remain a cause.

Note: women between the ages of 50 and 70 and men between the ages of 50 and 60 are most likely to develop depression. Here is an overview based on the German population of adults who suffer from depression each year[4]

---

[4] Busch, MA, Maske UE, Ryl L, Schlack R, Hapke U, the prevalence of depressive symptoms and diagnosed depression in adults in Germany. Federal Health Gazette - Health Research -
Health protection. 2013; 56(5):733-9

Age	Women who suffer from depression	Men who suffer from depression
18 to 29 years	5 out of 100 women	2 out of 100 women
30 to 39 years	7 out of 100 women	3 out of 100 women
40 to 49 years	9 out of 100 women	4 out of 100 women
50 to 59 years	11 out of 100 women	6 out of 100 women
60 to 69 years	11 out of 100 women	5 out of 100 women
70 to 79 years	6 out of 100 women	3 out of 100 women

Then, we want to take a closer look at the individual causes.

The genes

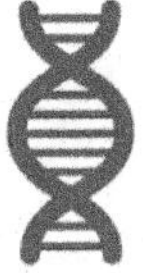 It is now undisputed that genes play a role. Depression runs more often in families; - if your parents have depression, chances are, so do you or so you will.

The probability of you suffering from depression as a result of inheritance is 15%! The genes indicate the probability, but nothing is set in stone. No gene can be "blamed" for. Accordingly, there is a particular gene constellation that plays a role. If you show that genetic constellation, it does not mean that you also have to suffer from depression. Rather, it is simply a risk factor that can lead to depression, although it doesn't have to.

Environmental influences

The environmental factor is now much more challenging to identify Everything that happens around you, what you consciously and unconsciously perceive, how you experience your environment, al of this is part of environmenta influences.

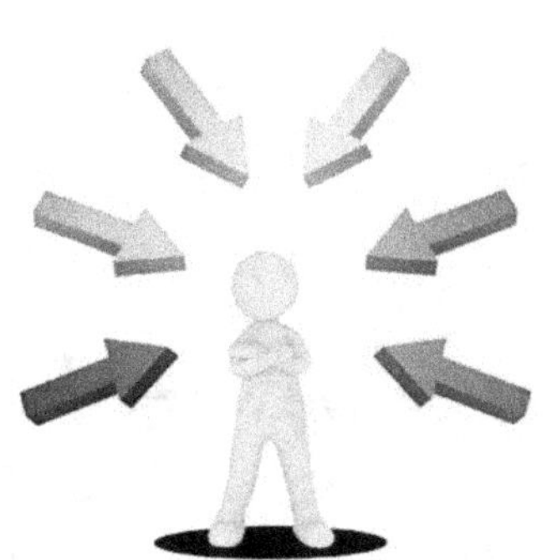

Imagine what a large area this has to cover! The environmental factors also include many individual experiences and events that you perceive in your environment. Starting with your childhood (how did you grow up, in which environment, etc.), your social life, your professional life.

All of these are environmental influences that shape you and promote or prevent the development of depression. Searching for environmental influences as a cause of depression is particularly like searching for a needle in a haystack! Not only is immense patience required here, but also a lot of research needs to be put into the causes. It is no wonder that psychotherapists do a great job when they go on that journey with the patient to take a closer look at environmental influences.

Environmental influences are all those areas that have an external influence on our lives and promote the development of depression.

Stressors

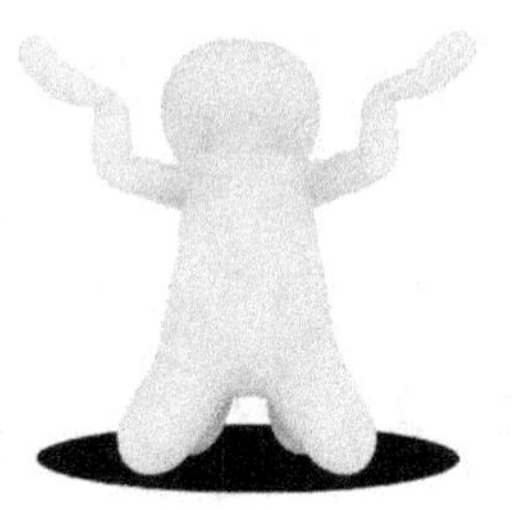

Today it is hard to imagine everyday life without stress. Stress is everywhere: at work, in private life, in relationships; stress is not on the side.

Rather, if you get into a permanent, even chronic stressful situation. then it gets dangerous, and the stress hormone axis comes into play. If you already carry a risk through your genes, then stress can undoubtedly cause depression to break out. The genes influence the hormonal balance in the brain. If it is disturbed, the stress hormone axis can change. The stresses hormones adrenaline, noradrenaline, and cortisol are increasingly released. The result is that you can no longer calm down. A "vicious cycle" begins, and constant stress leads to increased transmission of stimuli. However, since the brain's messenger substances are imbalanced, the stimuli are not transmitted correctly, influencing the stress hormone axis. The stress hormone axis then releases even more adrenaline, noradrenaline, and cortisol, and the cycle starts all over again!

Stress is also a cause that can promote depression. Increased stress can also make therapy more difficult. However, a distinction must be made here again. There is no such thing as a stress-free life. For a short time, stress is simply part of life. But the trick is to leave this stress behind. Only permanent, chronic stress leads to problems. As a rule, short-term stress is not a problem, but it can be the drop that brings the barrel to overflow and lead to depression in this case. If depression already exists, the person affected should urgently learn to cope with stress and, of course, stay away from permanent stress. While it can be said quite simply, there is a very strenuous learning phase in which the person affected should completely rethink their life and reduce stressful situations.

The following can be said: permanent or chronic stress promotes depression considerably. It becomes particularly critical when the genes are already doing some "preliminary work", and a certain imbalance already exists in the brain's messenger substances. On the other hand, brief stress does not trigger depression, but it can bring the barrel to overflow.

For more information on stress and stress management, you can find good, so-called eustress and bad, so-called distress, at our book homepage.

Psycho-trauma

Psychological trauma is a very special, sometimes complex, possible cause of depression. Psychological trauma is a situation that the brain cannot process. It most closely resembles excessive demands, to which the brain reacts with "psychological protective" mechanisms. Trauma can be experienced in many ways. Physical or emotional experiences of violence,, serious illnesses, loss, and neglect can cause trauma. Trauma can have psychological as well as physical effects. But what exactly happens?

For example, you hear someone die in a car accident right before your eyes. These experiences, impressions, and emotions can be so intense that it leads to an overload in the brain. It's a little like a light bulb burning out. But since the brain wants to protect itself, so-called protective mechanisms take effect. The experience is frequently subconscious, i.e., not accessible, processed, and stored for you. There is, therefore, a lack of memory. This particularly affects traumatic experiences in childhood. But that doesn't mean that the trauma has disappeared or been forgotten. It would be nice if it did not affect you. But that is not the case. And so, the profound experiences, memories, and emotions slumber in the deep expanse of your brain and break out every so often.

The brain is still unable to process what has been

experienced. The challenging thing about it is that trauma is usually unconscious and must be made conscious again through

targeted psychotherapeutic measures to deal with it. This is exactly where the danger lies. You know that something is wrong and that your reactions and feelings are too intense and violent. Let's stay with the example of the accident: For instance, you can have a racing heart, panic, sweaty hands, and enormous fear as soon as a car passes too close to yours without an obvious reason for this behavior. Traumatic experiences are therefore challenging to identify and therefore also to treat. However, this can lead to depression or another mental illness, the most common being post-traumatic stress disorder (PTSD). It is only plausible that overstimulation in the head does not pass the messenger substances without a trace. This can lead to an imbalance, which over time can trigger depression.

In summary, this means: If there is no professional processing your trauma, it can trigger depression or another serious mental illness. It is particularly important here that a disease such as PTSD is ruled out through the practitioner.

More on the subject of PTSD on our book homepage www.depressionenberwinden.de.

Biochemical changes

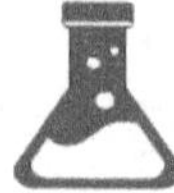

The biochemical changes can sometimes promote and trigger depression. The hormones serotonin and norepinephrine play an important role here.

Among other things, they are responsible for a positive mood. If there is an imbalance, the release of the stress hormone (cortisol) increases considerably and can be detected in the blood and urine. However, it is still unclear whether the biochemical balance is the cause or the consequence of depression. It is a bit like asking which came first: the chicken or the egg?

The fact is, however, that biochemical changes are associated with depression. Research on this is carried out diligently and is constantly being further developed.

Resilience

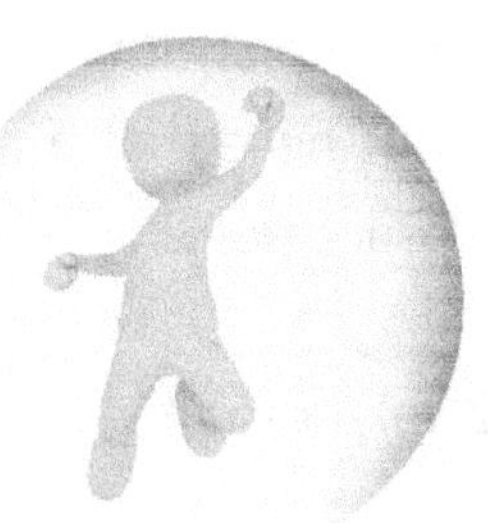

Resilience, also known as mental toughness, plays an essential role when it comes to depression. Resilient people, i.e. people with increased psychological resistance, are less likely to get depression, unlike those people whose resilience is less pronounced.

What is resilience all about? This refers to all the factors such as good crisis management and stress management skills, self-confidence and self-confidence, knowledge of one's strengths and weaknesses, and trust in one's skills and abilities. Resilience is not innate per se but has to be acquired through one's life. Conversely, this means that everyone can learn resilience. Less resilient people are more susceptible to mental illness, which includes depression. A lack of resilience can sometimes be a cause of depression.

Sleep disorder

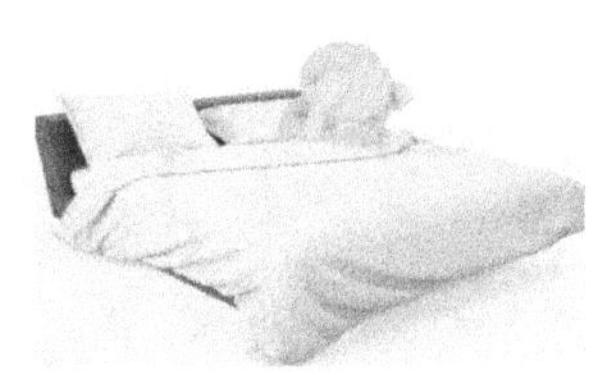

Similar to the biochemical changes, the same applies to sleep disorders. Sleep disorders can be described as both a cause and a symptom.

Sleep troubles include disturbed sleep phases and difficulty falling asleep and staying asleep, including waking up early and extreme lethargy during the day. Insomnia is not just a symptom of depression; it can also be considered the cause.
A chronic lack of sleep causes the brain's neurotransmitters to get mixed up, which means that this imbalance favors depression. Sleep disorders don't always have to turn into tangible depression. They can also trigger depressive moods. The hormone serotonin, which, among other things, regulates sleep, is responsible for both situations.

Pregnancy

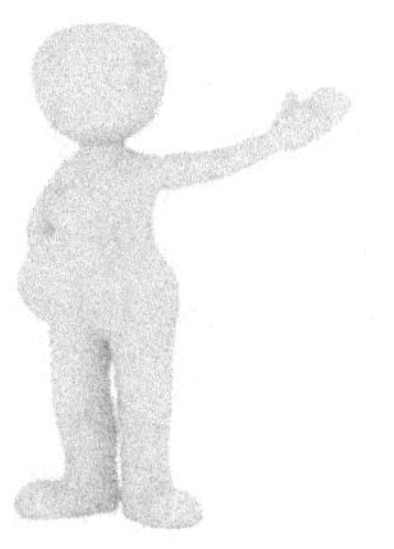

Much happens in the female body during pregnancy. It is a masterpiece phenomenon to create and carry new life. At no other time are so many hormones active in the female body as in pregnancy.

However, the hormonal thunderstorm in a pregnant woman's body can trigger depression. About 12 out of 10,016 pregnant women suffer from a so-called pregnancy depression, which can persist beyond childbirth [5].

In most cases, the end of depression is in sight after birth. In some cases, the depression can continue beyond pregnancy and does not go away within a few weeks of giving birth. In severe cases, psychotherapy and treatment with antidepressants have proven to be a good strategy for depression in pregnancy.

---

[5] www.bundesaerztekammer.de access 08.2020

Symptoms

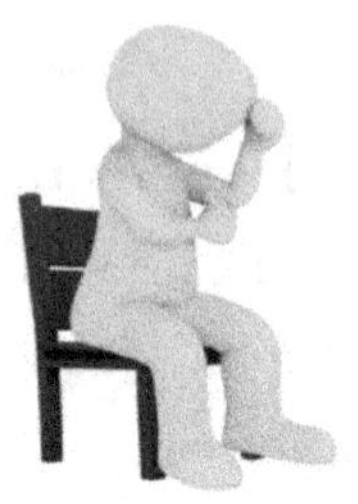

Around 12 out of 100 people in Germany suffer from depression at some point in their lives [6]. Among children and adolescents in Germany, 11 out of 100 under 18-year-olds develop depression.

The question remains open; how you can recognize depression? This is exactly where the symptoms come into play.

We have already got to know the 3 main symptoms of depression and the 7 secondary symptoms. In addition to these symptoms, it also comes to a range of other psychological and physical symptoms experienced by patients during the depression. The intensity and also the variety of symptoms are quite different and vary from person to person. Symptoms also depend on the severity of the depression. In most cases, the symptoms become more pronounced and increase in intensity as the depression progresses.

---

[6] Study "Current Health in Germany "(GEDA) 2014/2015
   8 BELLA study, a survey on the mental well-being and behavior of children and adolescents, 2009 to 2012

You already know that a depressed mood, inner emptiness, and listlessness are among the common symptoms of depression. Self-doubts, feelings of guilt, lack of concentration and attention, sleep disorders, restlessness, and the loss of sexual interest and desire are the lesser known symptoms. Those affected often complain of unspecific abdominal pain or headaches. The list of individual symptoms is long and very varied. Notice:

Main symptoms

- Despondency
- Loss of interes
- Letharg

In addition to these main symptoms, there are 7 other so-called secondary symptoms-- according to ICD, 10-- as of 2020:

- Difficulty concentrating and paying attention
- Declining self-esteem and   self-confidence
- Feelings of guilt, but also the feeling that they are no longer worth anything
- negative and bleak prospects
- Thoughts and intentions of suicide, including self-harm
- Sleep problems, difficulty falling asleep and staying asleep
- unwanted weight loss or weight gain

Secondary symptoms

Apart from the main and secondary symptoms, there is a list of symptoms that illustrate the first signs of depression. A lot of sensitivity on the part of the practitioner is required here because these symptoms can also represent other diseases.

Early symptoms include:

Early symptoms

- Non-specific pain, such as a headache or abdominal pain
- prolonged and lead tiredness, exhaustion, or severe lack of energy
- decreased sexual interest
- increasing listlessness, apathy
- Depressed and depressed mood
- Sleep disorders
- Loss of appetite or an increase in appetite

As you learned at the beginning of the chapter, more people get depressed as they get older. However, the symptoms express themselves a little differently in old age, or there are other clues to the symptoms already mentioned:

Additional symptoms

- Very pronounced tiredness and exhaustion
- severe weight loss
- physical pain
- Medical symptoms that cannot be classified
- memory problems
- social withdrawal
- Refusal of fluid and food intake - medication can also be refused
- Conflicts regarding personal care, no longer able to care for yourself
- Increased to extreme consumption of alcohol and sedatives

So far, we have not considered two groups of people: men and children. The symptoms can express themselves in differently in these groups. So, the first thing we want to do is show the symptoms of depression in men.Danger! Men suffer differently

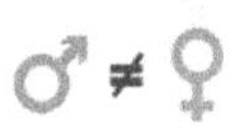

Depression is less obvious and common in men. There are different approaches to why depression affects women more often. On the one hand, the thesis is put forward that men suspected of having depression see a doctor less often and prefer to deal with the situation independently. On the other hand, the symptoms of depression in a man are different from the common symptoms. As a result, it is difficult for some practitioners to diagnose men correctly-- depression can remain undetected for a long time.

But what are the differences?

Men have different symptoms of depression than women. This does not mean that the three main symptoms can be ignored. These occur equally in men and women. It is now known in medicine that in many men, depression and aggression are closely linked. This doesn't mean that every man who gets depressed is automatically aggressive. But this connection is significant. The feelings of anger and discomfort play a major role. Depressed men often react very irritably and aggressively in situations where both emotional states play a role.

This circumstance is then associated with massive feelings of guilt. "Waves of anger" come over you. These express themselves psychologically, but above all physically: redness of face, sweating, accelerated heartbeat, dizziness, and tremors. A whole new worry naturally arises from these physical and psychological symptoms, namely the fear of total loss of control.

Symptoms specific to men

- Anger and discomfort
- exaggerated, aggressive reaction to "little things."
- Feelings of guilt
- Tantrums and waves of anger
- Waves of anger manifest themselves physically: flushed head, sweating, accelerated heartbeat, dizziness, and tremors
- Loss of control and worry about it
- irritability
- Often, men with depression, are resentful and quick to make many allegations
- Stress intolerance
- Increased to extreme willingness to take risks
- Socially conspicuous behavior (e.g., inappropriate behavior)

- Increased consumption of drugs, alcohol,
- Drugs and other addictive substances
- Dissatisfaction in all areas of life
- The constant fear of failure
- Feelings of guilt

These symptoms can, but do not have to, play an essential role in addition to the symptoms of depression mentioned. They often stand in the way of the classic idea of depression, as many people still assume that depressed people sit listlessly in the corner all day. Should you or a relative notice such symptoms in combination with the common symptoms, you should consult your family doctor or, as a relative, seek a conversation with the allegedly affected person. Pay attention to your loved ones.

Depression in Children

Recognizing depression in children and adolescents and then correctly interpreting the symptoms is particularly difficult. It's not because the symptoms and behavior are undetectable. Rather, they cannot be clearly distinguished from childhood development and puberty, so-called adolescence. This problem often is affected by the environment; in most cases, the parents should act upon detection.

How can we expect the people around them distinguish

characteristics of depression from the circumstances of adolescence and puberty when even trained professionals are sometimes unsure?

Depression in children and adolescents often expresses itself entirely differently. So, you can't lump all symptoms and irregularities together here. According to the German Depression Aid, dividing into appropriate age groups makes sense since the symptoms differ significantly. In the following, a distinction is made between toddlers (1-3 years), pre-school children (4-6 years), school children (6-12 years), and teenagers (13-18 years). Here too, the listed symptoms are in addition to the other symptoms.

Toddler

- Intense and frequent crying
- Expressionless face
- Increased irritability
- Brackets on caregivers
- Heavy sucking on the thumb
  - Weighing and rocking your own body
- Not interested in participating
  - No interest in gaming or pronounced gaming behavior
  - Problems eating, too much or too little appetite
- Sleep problems and abnormalities, difficulty falling asleep and staying asleep

Pre-schooler

- The depressed and sad expression on your face
- Reduced facial expressions and gestures
- Unstable in mood
- Shows no interest in participating, withdraws into himself
- Lack of interest in exercise
- Aggressive or refusing behavior
- Inner tension and restlessness
- Sleep problems and abnormalities, difficulty falling asleep and staying asleep
- Eating disorders, too much or too little appetite.

School-child

- Expressions of grief and sadness
- Difficulty concentrating
- memory problems
- Problems with school performance
- Fear, particularly of the future
- Feelings of guilt and strong self-criticism
- Inwardly withdrawn behavior
- Loss of feeling hungry
- Problems falling asleep and staying asleep

- Thoughts and expressions of suicide (not exclusively verbal, also often in pictures or with observing gaming behavior)
- Low self-confidence and increased self-doubt
- Fear
- Restlessness
- Difficulty concentrating
- Mood swings and   abnormalities

Teenager

- Performance issues
- The increased impression of not meeting social and emotional demands
- Social withdrawal and isolation
- Physical and psychosomatic abnormalities, such as headache and abdominal pain
- weight loss or increase
- Problems falling and staying asleep
- Thoughts, expressions, and attempts of suicide

In summary

Depression cannot always be identified at sight. The differences are far-reaching and often contradictory. People affected by depression are often dependent on their surroundings to react because it is not uncommon for those who are ill to know that there is depression behind it. Often, the symptoms are passed on to occupational or social stress; in old age, it is often assumed that these are age-typical changes. In doing so, these false assumptions turn out to be the beginning of a long and stony path of suffering. In this case, it is better to take a closer look, observe and act diligently.

The Diversity of Depression

If the symptoms are so varied and diverse, how do they affect the various forms of depression? Depression is not only one of the most common mental illnesses; but also has a diverse range of symptoms. Depression is assessed and diagnosed according to the "ICD-10 key", the "International Classification of Diseases." But these subject-specific subtleties are often unclear terms; bohemian villages. But it doesn't hurt that you get a rough overview of the diversity of the disease. Why is that important? Not all depression is created equal. Many different forms and symptoms unite under the umbrella term-- depression. There are depressed moods, depressive episodes, but also various depressive disorders. The following pages provide an overview.

Differential diagnostics

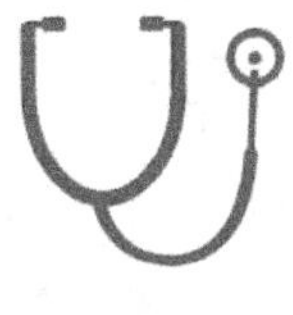 Of course, everything starts with a diagnosis. The doctor provides that. You already know the symptoms of depression. Of course, with such a symptom, the case is apparent, or perhaps not? It's not that simple.

Although a guess can be made relatively quickly, that doesn't mean that it is the correct diagnosis. If the practitioner is sure it is depression; he/she makes the so-called differential diagnosis. This is about excluding diseases that have similar, sometimes even the same symptoms. If these diseases can be ruled out using differential diagnosis, only one possible cause of the symptoms remains: depression.

With the wide range of depression, a differential diagnosis is particularly important to precisely determine the diagnosis. 3 differential diagnoses must be ruled out in the event of depression.

On one hand, there is dysthymia and, on the other hand, seasonal affective disorder. Not infrequently, however, depending on the symptoms, bipolar disorder is also an option.

Lots of technical terms! To save you a trip through medical dictionaries, we would like to briefly introduce you to the individual terms.

Dysthymia

Dysthymia describes a mild form of depression that does not meet the criteria for depression. Do you remember the 3 main symptoms and 7 secondary symptoms above? No? Then feel free to take a look again briefly before proceeding. Typically, dysthymia can best be described as a permanent "low" mood. It forms the first differential diagnosis of depression.

Seasonal affective disorder

As you may have guessed, this disorder is the so-called "winter depression". It is concerned with the occurrence of depressive symptoms exclusively in autumn and winter when the days are shorter and the nights grow longer. Seasonal affective disorder is the second common differential diagnosis to depression.

Bipolar disorder

Bipolar disorder is a mental illness that usually takes a severe and chronic course. It is best described as a manic-depressive disorder. Those affected experience a substantial change in mood in phases of varying duration (sometimes days or up to months). It alternates between manic (excessive elation) and depressive phases. During the manic phase, the affected people can pursue highly risky behavior because their emotional world and thought processes are characterized by overestimating themselves. Decisions made are regretted immediately after the manic phase has subsided, making amends difficult. This can put people in deep despair and cause a feeling of hopelessness in them. The latter can give the subsequent depressive phase a particularly severe course if there is no adequate professional treatment. Between joyous and deeply saddened, bipolar disorder plays out with a high-risk potential for the life of the person affected and the lives of others.

Schizoaffective disorder

Here it gets complex again. Depending on the initial symptoms, the schizoaffective disorder also belongs to the differential diagnoses. However, it is a little different. In addition to depression, the focus is also on schizophrenia. This is characterized by delusions and hallucinations. Manic and depressive phases accompany. Delusional does not only mean hallucinations, rather, it is the impoverishment of mania; depression. The megalomania, on the other hand, is a classic example of mania. Since mania and depression often occur together, you can safely imagine at this point how precisely this differential diagnosis must be carried out. Although a simplistic description of the schizoaffective disorder has been presented here, the consequences for those affected are far-reaching.

Final thoughts

The field of differential diagnostics is broad. The three differential diagnoses presented are only the most common. Of course, depending on the symptoms, many other differential diagnoses can be considered, such as tumor diseases. It is a highly complex subject, but you should have heard of it at least once! Your doctor is responsible for the diagnosis and the exclusion of differential diagnoses.

Depressed mood

Depressive moods can affect anyone at least once in a lifetime but it cannot be compared to depression. Although some symptoms of depression characterize depressed mood, it is not as pronounced as in depression. Therefore, it is not uncommon for people to speak of depression in common parlance, although it is not true. Unfortunately, the actual illness is considerably lessened and weakened by the everyday use of the term to the sick's suffering.

Depressive episode

The depressive episode describes the depression in a graduated classification. Here at least two of the three main symptoms and some secondary symptoms must be consistent for at least two weeks. Only then can it be considered to be depression or a depressive episode of the same extent according to the ICD definition.

From this depressive episode, other forms of depression can develop. In principle, however, the following applies to the three main symptoms and the secondary symptoms: the more symptoms there are, the more severe the depression. The following applies to the prognosis: the sooner depression is recognized, the better the treatment and chances of recovery. This does not mean that depression is incurable, but it can be strenuous to treat permanently.

Recurrent depressive disorder

A recurrent depressive disorder likely describes a depressive episode that has been reignited over and over again. This form of depression does not follow a time sequence. A depressive episode is followed by months, even years, in which the person affected is free of any symptoms. But then the depression comes back with the next depressive episode. This is incredibly difficult to cope with for the people suffering, and it is not uncommon for them to lack the ability to deal with it. The repeated flare-up of the depressive episodes limits people enormously in their life, especially in life quality. It is not uncommon for it to have professional and social consequences as well. Such people can only exercise their profession to a limited extent, but in some cases, it also means permanent loss of the profession. Partnerships and social contacts can also break as a result.

The more frequently this type of depression appears and returns, the more likely it is to recur. Fast, but above all, therapeutically targeted action is of the greatest importance here.

Adjustment disorder

When it comes to depression, it is not uncommon for the question to arise whether it is a depression or whether an adjustment disorder. Adjustment disorder is one of the symptoms of depression. However, it does not meet the criteria for depression; The decisive difference here is that a certain event preceded the illness. This is often the case when a loved one dies, and an adjustment disorder can also occur in the event of lovesickness or changes in the job. The symptoms usually go away on their own after six months at the latest.

However, one should not take a closer look because an adjustment disorder can develop into depression over time.

Chronic depression

Depression does not always have to take an episodic course. It can also be chronic. But there are some differences in the intensity and, of course, also in the course. This is how episodic depression runs in so-called

relapses which are perceived as violent and intense. A chronic depression, on the other hand, runs without the episodes, so it is constant and always present. However, the symptoms are not found in the same intensity or severity, as in a depressive episode. However, this does not mean that those affected by chronic depression suffer less.

The level of suffering cannot be compared, as the two forms

of depression are very different. Chronic depression is characterized by common symptoms, which must last for at least 2 years. Often, however, the problem with this form is that chronic depression is not often diagnosed. Believe it or not, even those affected do not know that despite the symptoms, they are suffering from some form of depression. It is rare for those affected to accept the symptoms of depression, which takes a chronic course. It doesn't make therapy any easier. It seems essential to us here that chronic depression is not explicitly listed in the German classification system.

Depression and other mental illnesses

Depression doesn't necessarily have to occur alone. It mostly occurs in combination with other mental illnesses. Here, too, the question of the chicken and the egg arises. For this reason, it is not always clear whether depression is the trigger for another mental illness or whether another mental illness is the cause of the depression.
Which mental illnesses co-occur with depression?

Very often, depression is mentioned together with anxiety disorders. Phobias, panic attacks, generalized anxiety disorder - depression often plays a role here. However, it becomes particularly significant when the anxiety disorder takes on a chronic, i.e. permanent state. Depressive symptoms can also occur in these illnesses.

Burn-out and, more recently, the so-called burnout syndrome

is also often diagnosed as depression. Stress and stressful life phases - both positive and negative - can lead to burnout or bore out. Although bore-out and burnout are opposed to each other, it does not mean that depression can be more or less excluded.

Depression can also co-exist with other mental disorders. In addition to mental illness, depression can occur together with physical illnesses.

This does not mean possibly causal diseases such as thyroid disorder, but the mentally stressful diseases such as cancer, heart attacks, etc. It can be difficult to distinguish it from the adjustment disorder. So, there is a multitude of combined possibilities in which depression is part of the diagnosis.

A far-reaching disease

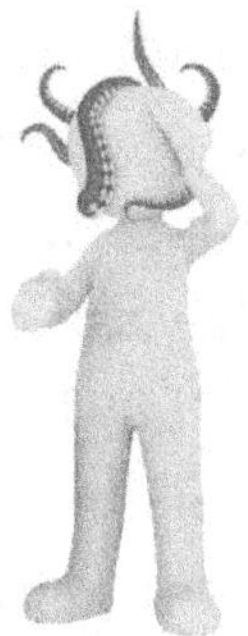 If you are or someone important to you is suffering from depression, then it means a lot of suffering for the person concerned and their relatives and caregivers. As a result, depression affects many areas of life.

Depression can indeed be described as a far-reaching disease. Do you remember the introduction? We wrote that some people would describe depression as an octopus that pulls them down into infinite black void with its mighty tentacles. This example can be used to picture how someone affected by depression is not surrounded by this octopus but carries it through life on its head or shoulders. The octopus's tentacles reach around the person, push their friends away and defend themselves with all their might so that people suffering from depression can hardly go about their everyday lives. It starts when you get up in the morning. You would like to get up. But the octopus sits on you, sucks itself tightly with its suction cups, and keeps you lying under the mighty animal; unable to defend yourself.

It is not an easy task to make the stages of depression clear and understandable.

Some different approaches and books try to convey this disease understandably. But it remains the same whatever octopus, dog, or an uncanny power: if the messenger substances in the brain are disturbed, and they can no longer carry out their work correctly and transmit stimuli, then you fight a hard fight against an invisible enemy! The following chapter will deal with the effects of this-- by no means hopeless-- struggle for those affected.

The Meaning of Depression

Note: Depression means something different for everyone!

No two people suffering from depression go through the same symptoms or struggles.

Although invisible to outsiders, depression is a serious illness. It is precisely because it is not visible, and those affected do not hobble, walk through the day on walking aids or wear a cast, that the general population often assumes that depression is not significant or real. Queuing, laziness, and other accusations must be endured. Finding the strength to get out of bed in the morning and face the day's challenges is the first hurdle that has to be overcome. But several other obstacles are awaiting the people suffering from depression. The smallest mistakes can bring everything to a standstill in everyday life.

So far, we have only talked about getting up in the morning. You didn't have to go to work, and the shopping hasn't been done either yet! Things that are completely normal, even banal, for healthy people can be an insurmountable obstacle for people suffering from depression. So much invisible hardship, and instead of help, there are often accusations and helpless statements from outsiders. We have listed a few examples to peruse below.

"Just smile!"

"You're pulling a face again today!"

"You just have to go out again!"

"Why are you hanging around like that?"

And bang! Even when well-meant, such statements do not help the patient. Instead, they alienate or isolate him.

First of all, it is not easy to do with depression. Second, pulling a face probably has more in common with an imbalance in the brain than with the other person wanting to pull a face! The life of someone suffering from depression has nothing in common with being left hanging! It is a daily struggle for survival on many fronts.

But what does it mean to be suffering from depression?

For the affected

How can you imagine that now? The following lines are sample descriptions from the affected point of view. Certainly, you have been hit badly with a cold before - so bad that you have barely made it out of bed. You were so physically and mentally exhausted that you immediately lie down again. Then when you woke up, it wasn't any better. You didn't care if your apartment looked like a pigsty or not. You needed rest and a lot of it! Every day feels this way with depression. But the terrible thing is that many days, weeks, months, and sometimes even years in the future will look like this! Your cold will subside after a short time, and you can resume everyday life but in the case of depression, nobody knows how long it will last.

The same goes for feelings. Many people have been bitterly disappointed at one point or another. This feeling eventually disappeared, and now the feeling is only a shadow in the memory. But for people with depression, those first moments are real. Over and over again, for day, weeks, months, and years they go through this disappointment. There's no fading; it's like a loop.

You certainly know the situation in which you have to decide and have these consequences for your future life. These are decisions that nobody likes to make, for fear of having made the wrong decision in the end and having to face the consequences. Healthy people can deal with it and find other solutions and strategies. However, people suffering from depression are caught in this uncertainty back and forth; yes, no--- with every little decision that has to be made. Banal things, for example: which socks should I wear today are real challenges for people with depression. No, living with depression is not an easy life!

Oh no, you are neither lazy nor do you consciously deny the activity. How much would you like to be a part of life? Getting up in the morning without any problems, drinking a coffee, and full of anticipation for the rest of your day.

Are you waiting for what the day may bring?
No, that is not the case. You're sick. You suffer from depression and struggle to get through it every day. Each day is darker than yesterday and much blacker than the next. Depression is awful, that's for sure!

For the environment

A lot has been said in this book about those affected. The environment, the next of kin, and the loved ones are often ignored. A fatal mistake, because depression affects not only the sick person but also the environment.
Relatives are often on hand with well-intentioned advice. But that advice, although well-meant, can sometimes be completely wrong in its effect.
You want to help the affected person because you appreciate and love that person. You want to be there for the person suffering from depression, you want to support them, and you often get caught in the clutches of depression yourself along the way. As is the case with alcohol, relatives can also become co-dependent. For this reason, relatives should distance themselves. For you as a relative, this means that you can and should be there for the sick person but not lose sight of your interests and needs.

But not all sufferers can hope for understanding. It is tough for relatives to understand this illness, and react to it accordingly. As a relative, you should, therefore, always keep in mind that it is an illness. The affected person does not wear rose-colored glasses, but black glasses, if at all, which distort their worldview and perception and reprograms them incorrectly. Be aware of this and avoid well-intentioned advice for the person concerned.

Most importantly, family members must know that they are not therapists. Dealing with people suffering from depression also means deep and massive cuts for relatives- the octopus will try to catch relatives too! Therefore, it can be constructive if relatives also get help from counseling centers or psychotherapy. The solution to the riddle is here, too: self-protection comes first!

For the job

The economy and depression are in serious conflict. However, the number of people suffering from depression has increased in recent years due to Misbelief. The statistics do not say that the number of people suffering from depression has increased, but that such people are more likely to seek help and thus have a good chance of recovery as part of therapy.

However, mental illnesses, including depression, are picking up speed and are now leading the way. The sick
leave days for mental illnesses are far ahead of those for

cardiovascular diseases, muscle or bone diseases, or respiratory tract diseases.

Additionally, everyone must be aware that mental illnesses are currently the main reason people have to retire early or suffer from a reduced ability to work[7].

This situation is a bitter pill not only for the economy but also for those affected. Well, not everyone with depression loses their job! So much should be said at this point. But too much pressure, incorrect handling of the disease, and delaying the depression lead to a relapse and cost the economy vast sums of money due to the lost/reduced workforce.

To quote numbers: mental illnesses cost the economy 15.5 to 21.9 billion euros annually, and the trend is rising [8].

The question remains why some branches of the economy get stuck with their conventional thinking. Why don't they adapt or encourage an evolving way of dealing with mental illness?

Fortunately, there has been a positive trend towards corporate health management in recent years. There are numerous examples in German companies that systematically promote the physical and mental health of the employees.

---

[7]German Federal Pension Insurance (2015). Pension insurance in time series. DRV fonts volume 22

8https://www.allianz.com/de/presse/news/studien/news-2011-04-13.html

Interestingly, the chicken and the egg question also arise here, as the interconnection between depression and the workplace is very intricate. While the workplace can certainly encourage depression, for example, if a genetic predisposition or a traumatic experience makes depression likely, the opposite situation can also be the case. Here, the workplace helps people suffering from depression to find their way back into their life, build up a structure, and consolidate their profitability. The question that arises here is how extensively people can contribute their creativity.

Either way, work, and depression have to be viewed individually on a case-by-case basis, and above all, professionally!

Understanding

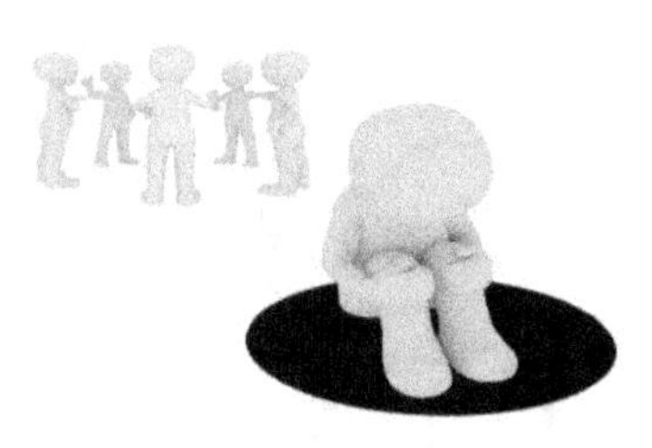

Many people suffering from depression report a lack of understanding within the social environment. Today, depression is becoming more and more socially accepted but it has not always been the case!

Not only depression, but also all other mental illnesses were for a long time divided into black and white taboo: either one could hide one's mental illness, or one was pushed to the outskirts of social life and treated as an eccentric or foreign body. (See also on our homepage for current book recommendations and reports on this.)

There has not been a comprehensive understanding amongst the general public for long. In many countries, these patients are still treated like in the Middle Ages! This understanding is still fragile!

Mental illnesses are not accepted by everyone. As if it wasn't already difficult enough for those affected to deal with the depression, they are often accused of being an actor, queuing up to get a little pity and attention, or just being lazy. You can imagine what such accusations trigger in those affected! They certainly do not contribute to a faster recovery. On the contrary!

So why is there not more understanding in such an enlightened society? This question can be answered quite easily. If the arm breaks, the injured person is given a cast which is visible. If you have a cold, your nose runs, coarse throat means to speak hoarsely, and to sneeze and cough. Puffy eyes and a pale face complete the visible symptoms.

Although depression can also have visible symptoms - for example, petrified and expressionless facial expressions - all the externally visible signs that show sickness are absent. Depression sufferers do not have a bandage around their head, they do not wear a cast, and they do not have a running nose. You won't find any crutches or puffy eyes with them. It is behavior that this disease affects. For too many people, unfortunately, the principle still counts at this point: what you can't see isn't there!

For example, there are also ancient views: "An Indian knows no pain.", or "What does not kill you makes you stronger!", Statements with fatal consequences for those affected! People with depression already feel down, suffer from self-doubt and self-reproach, and are also confirmed outside with such statements.

On the other hand, the question naturally arises about how relatives of those affected can understand the disease if they cannot understand the symptoms and effects. One thing is certain: the best description of the symptoms of depression can only begin to describe what those affected go through!
So, if you can empathize with the symptoms of depression, you have already suffered from depression yourself. However, this statement does not contribute to greater understanding of depression in itself!

Even though depression cannot be "seen" like a cold or a broken leg, it should be responded to with a similar understanding. Standards and requirements that are set too high often lead to exactly the opposite effect. Would it occur to someone to run a marathon with a broken leg? Common sense already tells you that this endeavor is pointless and dangerous to health, especially since nobody would start a marathon with a broken leg! And in this way, depression should also be shown understanding. So, what could that look like?

The first important step is empathy. Familiarize yourself with your illness or the illness of your loved one, and inform yourself about the form of depression! Based on the symptoms, a lot can become more understandable, although not necessarily more palpable. The soul of an affected person is sick! If you are suffering from depression, you should tell the people around you who are important to you.

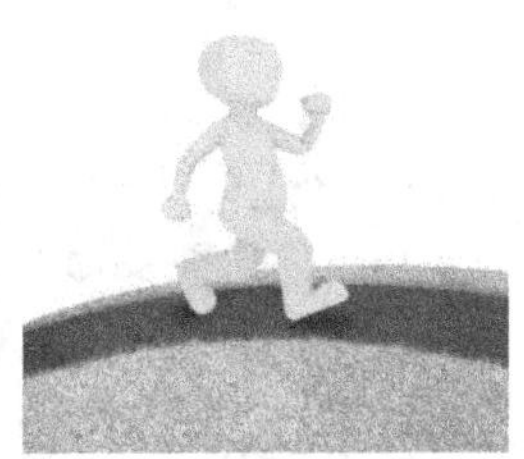

It is important that more understanding is shown. Relatives and friends should accept their loved one's soul is sick.

Although there is no runny nose or cough as a distinguishing feature, those affected should admit that it is tough for outsiders and healthy people to understand this serious illness. Therefore, the path of understanding for both sides is in the middle; everyone has to step towards each other, even if it is difficult!

Not a broken leg yet still restricted

Depression is protracted and can last for weeks, months, or even a lifetime. They influence an affected person's life and the life of the environment to a considerable extent. No matter how black the day is, at some point, there will be a small glimmer of light on the horizon, although you may not believe it at the moment!

Overall, dealing with the disease is a matter of perspective. Even when it is hard, hope should be maintained. Depression is an oppressive and serious illness of the psyche. It is characterized by hopelessness and helplessness among those affected and relatives. And yet, you can overcome depression and have another good morning!

Those affected are not to blame for the illness, nor did they cause it. It is a disease that comes again, but that eventually will go. The difference is in the duration. If the depression is viewed as such, support is given to the person affected and their relatives. A good therapeutic approach tailored to the severity of the person concerned is developed. The chances of recovery are very good.

The depression is not a broken leg, yet it limits a life in the same way, psychologically.

For Relatives

This chapter is written for relatives of people suffering from depression. Sometimes you can be overwhelmed, perplexed, and even helpless because you don't know how to connect with your family members; you neither know how to deal with the person concerned nor how to help yourself.

It's not an easy path. It has been marked by a lot of setbacks. Many relatives compare their situation with that of a hamster on a running bike: They try hard, kick themselves off, give everything, and it Is still not enough.

In doing so, many relatives are likely to lose track of their situation. The aim is that you can help the person concerned and support them in their recovery without breaking down at this task yourself! So how should you proceed? There are different ways you can influence your loved one/boyfriend/girlfriend's illness.

In this chapter, we would like to give you a few basic suggestions, ideas, and possibilities so that you, as a family member, get some basic required information.

The aim here is to ask how you can express your suspicions if you think that a relative or a person in your environment seems to be suffering from depression. Also, we will give you a few facts on how to deal with depression and how you can help yourself and your loved ones out of this. You also have to protect yourself a little bit. How this works will also be part of the chapter. So, let's start!

How should I make guesses?

Do you suspect that someone close to you may have had depression? Then you have already cleared a huge hurdle with your attention, and we would like to congratulate you! It is not uncommon for relatives to misunderstand and overlook the first signs. So, it takes a lot of sensitivity and good powers of observation to get the early signs correct to interpret. But what happens next? What are the right steps?

If you have the suspicion that someone close to you is suffering from depression, you can and should address the person directly. However, it is a question of the way, so: How do I appropriately address the person who is probably affected?
You should communicate your suspicions. Statements that could be formulated in this way or in a similar way will help you here:

I have noticed that you have been withdrawing a lot lately. You have always been interested in XYZ (interest of the person concerned) and talked about it with pleasure. That is different now. Am I correct?

You've been pulling back a lot lately, and I've seen you look down. I worry about you!

Your joy seems to have been lost. That makes me think a lot. I would like to do something about it with you. Is there something we can do together?

You seem unique to me. Lately, you seem to lack your zest for life. Would you like to talk to me about it?

As much as you want to be active immediately, you should always be careful to communicate your concerns about the person. You should urgently try to encourage yourself to avoid doing so.

These can, albeit be well-intentioned, put the affected person under a lot of pressure, and the shot could backfire. Such statements include, for example:

Let's just go out again.
Come on; we're going away for the weekend. Just get out and breathe fresh air.
Laugh again at last. Laughter helps!
That will pass if you do something about it now!

You cannot go the hard road for the depressed person. You can accompany the person, offer him / her help and observe.

What you can do to deal with the disease

If you have now found the beginning and could express your concerns to the person concerned, then the second step follows. The point here is that you offer help to the person suffering from depression. Communicate clearly, in this step, that you are willing to walk this difficult path together with the person, but you cannot replace a therapist! Encourage the person to make an appointment with the family doctor or specialist in psychiatry and psychotherapy (a neurologist is also possible).

 In some cases, however, the person concerned may be so affected by the depression that they cannot act or organize the appointment themselves. Here you can take on this task if the sick person so wishes.

In some rare and extreme situations, however, you may also need to call the emergency doctor. This is the case when the depressed person expresses suicidal intent. The emergency doctor can then arrange for you to be referred to a psychiatric facility as quickly as possible. Without wanting to arouse fears in you, it is a fatal mistake to believe that people who announce suicide will not commit.

We have already mentioned many manners to you in this chapter. Well-intentioned attempts at encouragement and general advice should be avoided. Instead, try to talk to the person concerned. Make an effort to understand

and avoid pushing the person too hard. Otherwise, it would only put the affected person under more pressure.

You already know that depression is a serious mental illness and that a person who has never suffered from depression cannot even imagine living with such an illness; that is quite normal too! You don't have to empathize with the illness to help the person affected. Because for people not suffering from depression, there is no way to empathize with these burdens. But you can understand the disease. After all, you also understand someone who has just broken a leg in an accident.

Ten ideas for dealing with those affected

You want to help the person who is depressed. That is more than just understandable and commendable! After answering the questions what is depression, how.

When they express themselves and what the chances of therapy are, relatives and friends are usually very interested in providing help to the person affected. The ten ideas should deal precisely with this: How can you help? What needs to be considered, and to what extent can help be offered? These following points should set you!

As much as you worry, you can't care too much for the sick person. It is alleviating for the suffering person to enjoy some independence. But that doesn't mean that you have to receive payment?. Make sure you are there for the person when he or she needs you.

1. Priorities

Focus on the things in life that are important. You should not judge the behavior of the sick person too personally either. It is essential: Set yourself specific priorities! Do not lose yourself in helping the other.

2. Take care of yourself

As much as you worry, you don't need to give the sick person too much care. It is better to give the sick person as much independence as possible. But that doesn't mean that you have to or should withdraw. Make sure you are there for the person when he or she needs you.

3. Take your time

Give yourself and the sick person the time they need to cope with the disease, especially in acute phases. Although one is inclined to accelerate the matter, you should instead take the small steps and enjoy small successes together with the person concerned.

4. Don't expect too much

No two days are the same. Therefore, keep adjusting your expectations. Overstrain and overstimulation do not help the sick person or yourself!

5. Set small goals

The goals should be realistically attainable for the sick person. Remain factual and communicate this without emotion. Again, think in small steps and take as much pressure off as possible. Celebrate the goal achieved.

6. Don't be offended

Remember that the sick person will tell you that they do not want to anger or vex you with their behavior. Depression is the expression of coping with one's experience. It's not easy, but certainly not directed against you!

7. Do what you can

Although depression often seems to affect almost every area of life, there are still "healthy" areas. Instead of focusing on what was currently paralyzed by the depression, you should concentrate together with the person affected on the areas in life where things are still going well and strengthen them

8. Stay calm

Even if it sometimes seems unbearably difficult, you should acquire a calm attitude towards life.

It will not only become more bearable, but also easier. Make sure you leave space for your feelings and emotions and deal with them consciously.

9. And what about medication?

Although the sick person may depend on medication, it is a matter between him/her and the doctor. Of course, you only want the best for your loved one/boyfriend/girlfriend and therefore pay close attention to whether the medication has been taken? But that's not your job! Don't feel responsible for it, nor should you put pressure on the person.

10. Be binding.

Keep appointments; appointments with the sick person, or postpone them if there is no other way. Make out beforehand that it is ok if he/she calls you at night or only the next morning, but appointments may not be postponed if there is "no desire," etc.

Recommendations and further instructions are on our homepage:

11. **Avoid co-illness**

You take care of your loved one or friend with great sacrifice. Yes, you would sacrifice it all for them, but you still shouldn't forget yourself. Don't get over-involved in a co-illness and then get sick yourself! You will have achieved nothing and, above all, hurt yourself.

A co-illness happens gradually, and thus it is not always immediately recognizable. So, you should be able to set limits and not wait until your batteries are completely exhausted! A very important aspect is that you continue to pursue your interests, live out your hobbies, and maintain social contacts. (note the ideas from the previous chapter!)

Self-help groups for relatives

Sometimes, however, it can also help and be pleasing if you participate in self-help groups for family members. You can also find links to this on our homepage.

In these self-help groups, the exchange of experiences is in the foreground, and you will quickly notice that you are not the only person far and wide who carries such loads on your shoulders! You should ensure rest - take undisturbed time just for yourself and do something good for yourself!

If you notice that you are overwhelmed with a situation, then you should by no means dismiss it as a short-term phase. Respond to it and seek appropriate help immediately. The family doctor can be the first point of contact, but charitable institutions can also provide you with extensive advice on this.

Find out more on the homepage of your city. The first contact points are often listed there under the health section. We have created a small overview of this on our homepage.

A Way Out of Depression

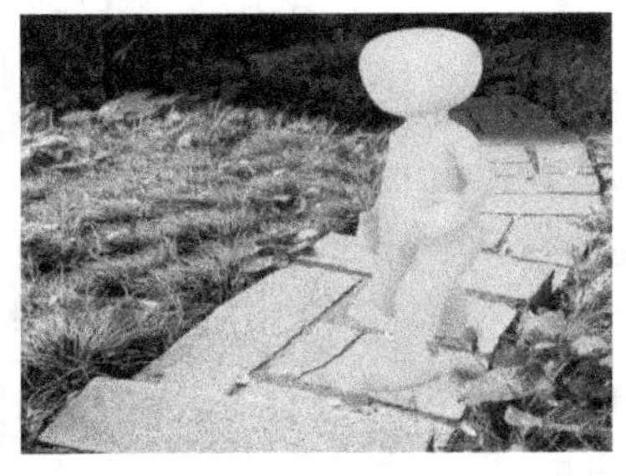

We would like to start by saying the good news: most depression cases can be cured! The sooner they are treated, the more likely a cure is! However, many types of depression do not go away on their own.

The affected person must therefore take action and seek professional help. The practitioner works with the person affected to find a way out of the depression. For this purpose, the diagnosis is at the beginning. First of all, depression must be precisely determined, both as a clinical picture and in terms of severity. Various therapeutic approaches are then discussed. In most cases, it is a combined therapy consisting of medication and psychotherapy.

However, how exactly each therapy looks in detail is very individual and therefore different from case to case.

There are good and bad days on the way out of depression. So, you will come across days on which you see no point in therapy and would like to break it off. But there will also be days when hope will return that you can overcome the illness and return to your everyday life.

This chapter is about the possible ways out of depression. For this purpose, we explain the current various therapeutic approaches. We would also like to explain to you what therapy means and what goals a therapist pursues. Since there are very many different opinions and views on the chances of recovery from depression, we also look at the prognosis and statistics. This chapter is intended to encourage you to walk the path out of depression.

Therapeutic approaches

There are several combinations of options that enable a stable passage out of depression.

Unfortunately, many therapeutic approaches are still full of prejudices from the general population. Although psychotherapy is much more widely accepted today than 20 or 30 years ago, patients often struggle with social prejudices! But it would help if you didn't let that deter you—the same counts for therapy with medication. Science and medicine have made tremendous advances in the last few decades, and medicines have been fine-tuned and made more efficient. A much more targeted dosage is possible nowadays, which means that the side effects can be kept within limits. The prejudice that one becomes a remote-controlled robot has long been outdated and no longer corresponds to the current picture.

Therefore, you should pay little attention to all these prejudices, preliminary opinions, and false information and instead focus on your recovery! Now that a little fear has made its way out of you, we would like to explain the various therapy options applicable to depression! We very much hope that you will have a better overview by the end of the chapter!

Medical therapy

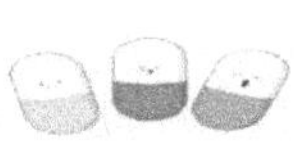 Depression is usually treated with something called an anti-depressant.

This is a drug that is used regularly and must be taken over a certain period of time to develop its full effect. As a rule, antidepressants take about 2-4 weeks (sometimes 6) when taken daily before noticing relief from the depressive symptoms. The onset of the effect depends, among other things, on the daily prescribed dose and the severity of the depression. However, the assumption that antidepressants should be discontinued without authorization as soon as an improvement is felt can be fatal. Depression may return with a vengeance, and drug therapy must be restarted. Therefore, discontinuation should only be discussed with the practitioner instead of opting out yourself. As a rule, antidepressants are taken for a further 6-12 months after the patient is symptom-free. This is used as prophylaxis and should prevent a relapse

But how do antidepressants work?

Antidepressants act directly on the brain. At this point, you remember the imbalance of the messenger substances. Many antidepressants prevent the messenger substances from being transported away in the synaptic cleft where they block the exits. This means that there are more messenger substances in the synaptic gap that can then transmit a stimulus.

In principle, the side effects of antidepressants are varied. Often, these occur primarily in the dosing phase, over a period of time.

It is therefore important that you consult your practitioner closely about this at the beginning. To avoid them, always read the package insert and ask your doctor or pharmacist if you are unsure. This is a preparation that best suits your life situation and needs. Sometimes it is also necessary to choose another antidepressant in an intolerance because, as with dress sizes, no one size fits every person.

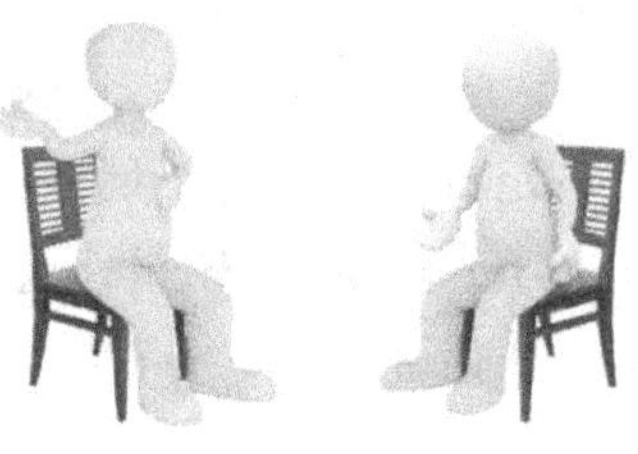

Psychotherapy

Psychotherapy offers a special and particularly successful form of therapy for depression in many ways. But what is it all about?

Psychotherapy is a form of therapy used to heal mental illnesses. Various procedures, techniques, methods, and approaches are pursued within psychotherapy. Psychotherapy can be carried out on an outpatient or inpatient basis. In outpatient psychotherapy, there is the option of a few sessions (usually 3-5, so-called probatory sessions) to decide whether a relationship of trust can be established between the patient and the practitioner. This is very important for successful therapy. Nobody likes to talk to someone with whom the "chemistry" is wrong.

In addition to getting to know each other, the type of psychotherapy is also decisive. At this point, you can imagine that there are many different forms of therapy and that each practitioner has a focus. In the case of depression, 3 procedures are possible, one of which is currently not reimbursed by the statutory health insurance companies. On one hand, behavior therapy and psychotherapy based on depth psychology must be mentioned; on another, humanistic psychotherapy. Since these forms are often used in therapy against depression, we would like to introduce them to you briefly.

Behavioral therapy

Behavioral therapy has operant and classical conditioning at its center. Both are stimulus-response models. To make it easier for you to understand: If you operate the door opener and touch the door handle, you will get an electric shock. Since the electric shock causes you to be in pain, you will no longer touch the door handle and the door opener at the same time in the future. You have learned that a combination of these two touches leads to pain. Behavioral therapy is specifically about recognizing and analyzing behavioral patterns and embedding new behavioral patterns. Behavioral therapy is not only about integrating new behaviors, but also about self-help. With the patient, new ways are sought in which the affected person can help themselves in difficult situations.

The basic premise behind behavioral therapy is simple: behaviors and patterns that have been learned can also be unlearned again. Over time, behavioral therapy has been broken down into many different approaches and models, each with its areas of focus to help patients.

Psychotherapy based on depth psychology

Behavioral therapy is opposed to depth psychology. In-depth psychology, the basic assumption is based on psychoanalysis. Depth psychology is about analyzing the psychological processes and experiences. Much can be deduced from the words-- depth psychology.

In this therapy, which usually lasts longer than behavioral therapy (sometimes years), the aim is to dive into the subconscious and make wishes, motives, and conflicts surface to the conscious level.

Moreover, depth psychology assumes that most of the damaging influences come from childhood and adolescence. If these two aspects are combined, you go on a journey through time into the unconscious of your own soul and see the causes for the current mental illness. The therapist and the patient work together to resolve the causes.

Depth psychology focuses less on changing behavioral patterns than on the clarification of unconscious conflicts, some of which may have been decades ago.

Humanistic Psychotherapy[9]

Humanistic psychotherapy (HPT) is a holistic procedure that enjoys growing popularity as an alternative to the previous forms of therapy. The HPT focuses on psychological growth through the activation and development of human resources (potentials). The aim is to be able to lead a meaningful, self-fulfilling and authentic life. From the therapist's perspective, a human's concept is based on the patient's resources, especially in regards to creating growth and constructive change. In the HPT, people are seen holistically.

One of the basic ideas of the HPT is that the human being already has the resources necessary for liberation from psychological suffering. The therapist and patients are tasked to find these resources, activate them, and apply them to life's problems. People's ability to be creative and self-reflective allows people to develop and shape their own lives throughout their lives.

In HPT, it is vital to ask the health insurance company in advance to what extent humanistic psychotherapy costs can be reimbursed. HPT is well established in many other countries, but most German statutory health insurances do not regularly cover the costs for this.

---

[9] After the text "What is Humanistic Psychotherapy?" Accessed 08-2020 by Werner Eberwein at http://aghpt.de with the kind permission of the author

You can find a link to the therapist and clinic search for outpatient or inpatient psychotherapy, as well as a video about the various techniques within HPT for depression on our book homepage:
www.Depressionenüberwinden.de.

All forms of therapy can demonstrate promising results. Behavioral therapy and psychotherapy based on depth psychology are the two procedures reimbursed in Germany by statutory and private health insurance in the event of a corresponding illness. You have to find out for yourself which form of therapy is suitable for you because everyone is different, and not everyone gets along equally well with one or the other form of therapy! The most sensible step is to seek advice from your practitioner in advance if you are unsure about the form of therapy.

Support groups

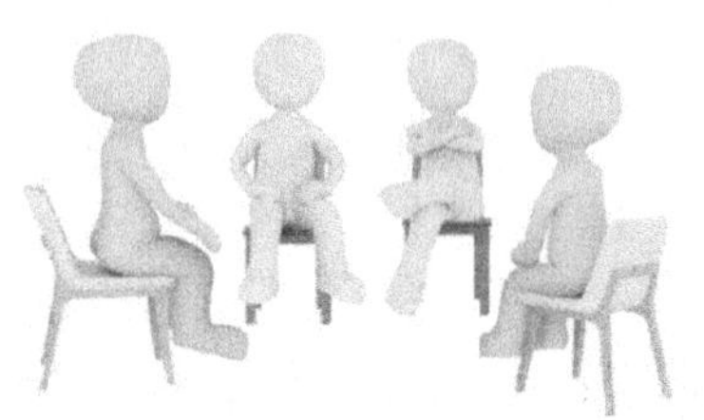

Self-help groups, under professional guidance, have also proven to be particularly effective. They work well in the case of addictions such as alcohol addiction but also for depression, as long as you get involved.

The advantage of a self-help group is obvious. The person suffering from depression moves into an environment where a group of people shares or shares the same fate: fight against depression. Nobody needs to explain themselves within the protected space because every participant knows how overwhelming depression feels. Usually, good exchanges can take place, and mutual solutions can be found. Those affected can also benefit from other people's experiences and thus have an enormous treasure trove of individual experiences in the fight against mental illnesses that they can fall back on.

But knowledge of the suffering from the disease brings with it a new bond with a lively exchange and a social life! Both are important steps in mastering the way out of depression.

Be careful! With all the advantages that a self-help group may bring, it should not be understood as psychotherapy or even a replacement. Alas, a support group is not for everyone and one should not be forced into it, even if only the best intentions may be behind it. A self-help group can be very positive for other forms of therapy if you want to and can get involved. If you don't want to go to the first meeting alone, please ask one of your friends, we are sure they will be happy to assist. For some groups, you can also register in advance, and someone will be on hand on the first evening for further questions.

You can find which self-help groups there are in your area and other helpful links on our accompanying website or the homepage of your city/district:
www.depressionenüberwinden.de.

Relaxation techniques

Various relaxation techniques can help the sufferer overcome thoughts and help with depression.

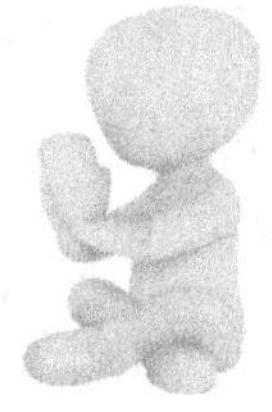

But what do these relaxation techniques involve?

The common relaxation techniques include progressive muscle relaxation and also autogenic training. However, these are not the only ones.

These relaxation techniques that can be used are just the most popular methods. In principle, what is good is allowed. Breathing exercises can be extremely beneficial for one person, while another finds absolute relaxation while painting or yoga.

Other techniques: color in mandalas, fill in crossword puzzles or meditation.

The variety of possible relaxation techniques is vast. Therefore, it is recommended that people suffering from depression and their relatives search together or individually and see what is suitable for them. In most cases, the various options have to be tried several times to form an opinion. Above all, only you can decide whether a type of relaxation technique helps you.

Incidentally, sport is often counted as part of relaxation. The fact that exercise and sport are good and important for depression is absolutely out of the question. However, relaxation techniques are about consciously coming to rest! An additional sport or exercise program can counteract depression very well!

You can find an up-to-date overview of other techniques on our book homepage.

www.depressionenüberwinden.de.

What other therapy options are there?

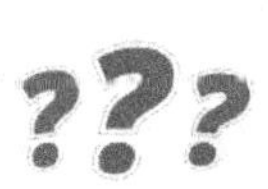

Of course, the therapy options with the approaches mentioned here are far from exhausted. There are many other ways.

Electroconvulsive therapy

Electroconvulsive therapy, or ECT, has proven itself apt in severe depression. Short electrical impulses are set in the brain under anesthesia, triggering a seizure in the patient. Thanks to anesthesia, there is only a brief thunderstorm in the head which is often unnoticed. How exactly ECT works is still unknown today. However, it is assumed that different brain regions that have been changed by depression interact. Incidentally, the effectiveness of ECT has been very well proven by various studies and is mainly used when the usual treatment attempts have failed, and the depression does not give way.[10]

[10] http://www.psychiatrie.med.uni-goettingen.de/de/content/patienten/243.html,Zugriff08-20

Vagus nerve stimulation

According to the latest studies, targeted nerve stimulation (vagus nerve stimulation) using electrical impulses is extremely effective against depression. Although these findings are still confined to German studies, this treatment has already been approved in the USA. The successes from the USA are impressive. Around 60% of people suffering from depression reacted to the treatment within 30 months to vagus nerve stimulation and were able to find their way back to normal life despite the worst prognoses.[11]

Animal Assisted Therapy

Animal-assisted therapy can also achieve success. However, since this is very special and requires that the patient is not afraid of the animal in question, it is not as widespread in its use. The animal, under favorable conditions, can help the person affected to return to normal life. Dogs and horses are mostly suitable for animal-assisted therapies. Cats, rabbits, and chickens are also used more and more frequently. The healing bond that is established with the animal is in the foreground.

---

[11]Psilocybin with psychological support for treatment-resistant depression: an open-label feasibility study, Robin L Carhart-Harris et

al

Psychedelic Therapy

According to the studies, the hallucinogenic mushroom extract is also currently being researched, and the primary results are promising. However, they are currently not approved as a therapy method outside of studies. Therefore, the therapy is mentioned here only for the sake of completeness and as an outlook into the future. Should there be any new findings, we will report them in one of the following editions or on our book homepage: www.depressionenüberzüge.de.

Self-therapy with these substances is not recommended under any circumstances. If someone offers you, we strongly advise against it, and instead, you should rather talk to your practitioner.

Light therapy

If you suffer from depression, the course and intensity is related to the dark months. Light therapy as an additional form of therapy could be correctly used. After waking up, the patient is exposed to a special light source for about half an hour, within a time frame of approximately 3 weeks. Before using this form of therapy, the doctor treating the patient should have contraindications (previous illnesses or even increased sensitivity of the eyes, condition after eye surgery, diabetes mellitus). You can find recommendations and ideas for daylight alarm clocks and their use on our website.

Goals of therapy for depression

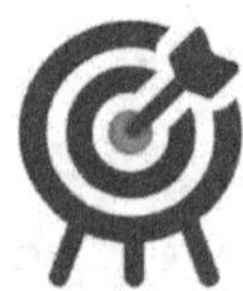 Essentially, the goal of therapy is the recovery of the sick person. Although depression is a well treatable disease, there are always exceptions.

In this course of the disease, therapy aims to alleviate the symptoms and thus improve the condition.

Basically, within the various therapeutic approaches, possible ways of stabilizing the patient and strengthening their resources are sought. In this way, the sick person should be given a new quality of life. Above all, though, is the feeling of not being at the mercy of illness anymore and to counter it. Since there are always days with depression when things worsen, you and your practitioner set the goals individually and sometimes very spontaneously. For example, on a bad day, the goal might be a positive one to describe the moment. On better days, you can set your first future goals and work towards these goals. The aim is that the person suffering from depression can return to completely normal life at the end of the therapy, participate in social and cultural life, and retake a life-affirming attitude.

Ultimately, in almost all therapies, the individual goals are formulated together with the patient. Progress can only be made if these suit the person. Hope, courage, and confidence are often the focus here.

What can I do?

When it comes to the way out of depression, initiative is required. Depending on the severity of the illness, this initiative is usually very individual.

Depending on the severity and impact of the depression, those affected and their relatives have several options to intervene themselves. That is why in this chapter, we would like to show you the various approaches and possibilities that you can do yourself to get through this phase of your life well. Since there are different measures, we distinguish this chapter between people suffering from depression and their relatives.

What can I do if I have depression myself?

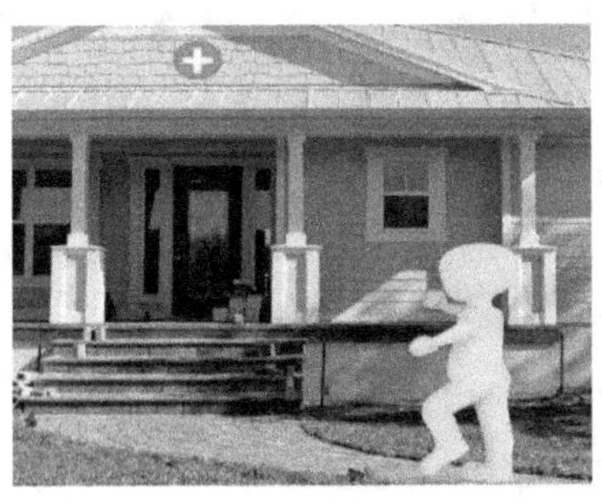

What you can do about depression depends on your symptoms and the course of your depression.
The first and most important step you should take is to see your GP.

If you like, a person you trust can also come. This offers a great advantage: if you cannot express yourself accurately, the person you trust may better describe your behavior.

When you have taken this step, the general practitioner will refer you to various specialists and initiate various therapies. You are particularly in demand here! You can significantly influence the therapy and thus the chances of recovery through the little things. For healthy people, it's little things! For you, as an affected person, there are sometimes giant hurdles.

Air and movement

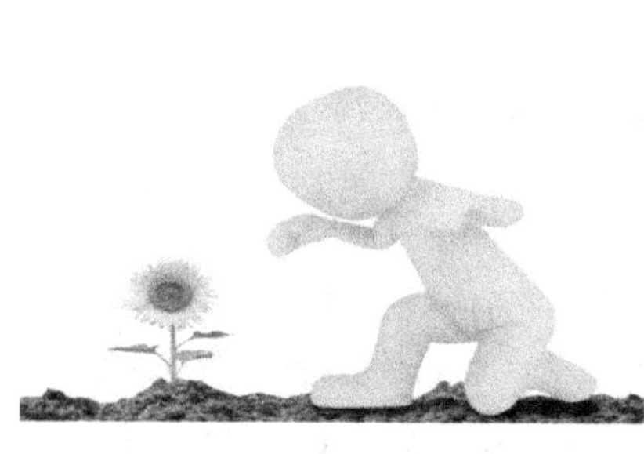

Depression does not like fresh air and exercise. Be uncomfortable! No, it does not have to be a high-performance sport, rather any light form will do. A walk, regularly around the familiar lap around the block is enough to improve your health considerably.

Since exercise is a miracle cure for depression, regularity is important here. Exercise every day if possible.

Do something! / Pleasant activities

Another way to stop depression is to do activities that neither overwhelm you nor undermine you. How about you paint mandalas? You are also welcome to call a friend and have a phone call with them. Short messages do not count here. If you have a better day with your illness, then go to the hairdresser or cook something good for yourself. You will be amazed at the good it will do you!

Structure time

Pull yourself up; that sounds so simple and natural. In healthy times it is easy! You get up and do the things that needed to be done. But with depression, the world is viewed with a tainted glass. It will undoubtedly take a while before you can go through your life in your old shape again. But you can already take the first small steps yourself. Make a weekly schedule of things you want to get done. You don't have to do witchcraft. Wash the dirty dishes on Mondays and open the letters on Tuesdays. Create a weekly plan based on your assessment.
You can find a form to fill out and an app to remind you on our book homepage.
www.depressionenüberwinden.de

When it gets darker, turn on a light

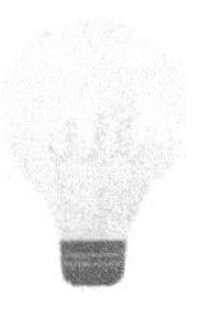

When the thoughts recirculate, you seem to be empty. Notice that you should intervene and do something e.g., breathing exercises, listening to your favorite music or take a soothing bath by candlelight!

Choose something that makes you feel good and hold something bright against the looming darkness —the point here is not to suppress the depression but prevent it for as long as possible. Over time, you will get better at finding what can help you. On our book homepage, you will find a list of suggestions for pleasant activities to download.

Nutrition

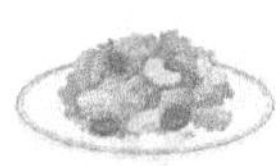 By the way, you can also influence depression with your diet. For this, you should eat a balanced and healthy diet. Eat lots of fresh fruits and vegetables, eat healthy fats and make sure you have enough protein.

But also treat yourself to a small piece of chocolate or some other treat if you feel like it. Don't overdo it with treats! A piece of chocolate can be eaten as a reward or as dessert, not for filling for the inner emptiness. Frustration eating can become a problem for many sick people and does not make things any better in the long term. Easier said than done; we know that but you can help yourself a little here by not buying anything sweet or salty when shopping and not hoarding anything in the house. Make yourself a meal: plan for the next week or a list for your next purchase. Maybe you always wanted to try a certain food.

Why not take advantage of the moment and get a cookbook with Greek, French, Indian cuisine and try everything once?

Make sure you are drinking enough fluids and drinking plenty of water. Indeed, there are studies on the subject. Decreased fluid intake can lead to depression[12]. On the other hand, you should eat alcoholic drinks and drinks with a lot of sugar dispense.

On our book homepage, you will find further information, including cookbook recommendations and a link to the calculator about how much fluid you need on average with your age and weight.

---

[12]Haghighatdoost F, Feizi A, Esmaillzadeh A, et al. Drinking plain water is associated with decreased risk of depression and

What can I do for a depressed person?

Relatives also have to help themselves! No, you do not suffer from depression, and you are sure to be happy about it. Yet, you shoulder a lot in this difficult time and even have to grow beyond your strength.

Such pressures are not a problem for a short time - after all, life would be boring if it weren't for turbulent times. But such a short phase can quickly develop into a permanent one! It is difficult to draw the line, especially when one is sick.

Family tends quite close to the person. But that's why you should pay attention from a healthy distance. This does not mean that you should leave the sick person to himself! On the contrary, you shouldn't sacrifice yourself either.

But what can you do for yourself now?

Recommend professional help

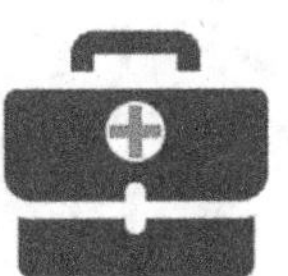 First of all, you should encourage the sick person to begin therapy and seek professional help. This project leads to a great burden.

In some cases, various therapies plan to involve the relatives. It is highly recommended to take advantage of this offer. You will find out more about the disease and how you can better deal with it. In many cases, there are also relatives' talks.

Here you will be informed about the sick relative's current status if they have agreed, and you can also get rid of the frustration.

Many relatives sooner or later, think that the demotivated behavior is directed towards them. You should bear in mind that it is the illness that speaks instead of your loved ones or friends. To be able to differentiate here, depending on the symptoms, is not easy. In conclusion, you cannot take everything personally!

If you have read this far, you have already taken this important step.

Be yourself!

Depression is an illness that can have wide implications, and that means over time the illness can affect you. For the benefit of the person concerned, for example, you do without your sport, regular visits to the theater, or a cozy evening with friends. Or maybe you feel guilty because you can experience joy and fun and the other person doesn't or cannot the same way. It would help if you pursued these activities instead. Take part in social life and have fun! So, you don't run the risk of your energy reserves being exhausted at some point.

Remove time pressure

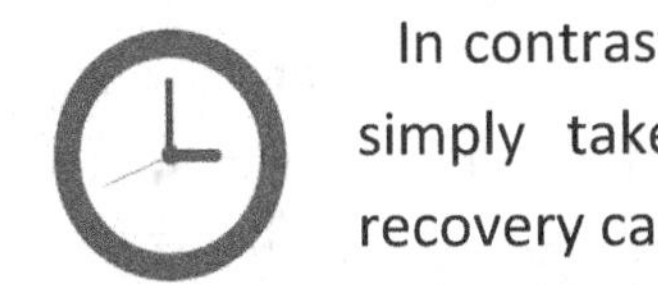

In contrast to a quickly cured cold, depression simply takes a lot more time. Usually, the recovery cannot be made out in advance. Therefore, you should plan generously and allow the treatment a lot of time, true to the motto: good things come with time. If you give yourself a generous time frame, you will also have less disappointment to deal with.

Once again: take care of yourself!

As much as you plan not to lose sight of yourself and not devote yourself to the person until you are exhausted, reality often shows a different face. We have many relatives who often end up completely exhausted and helpless.

Sometimes, you are also more prone to a mental illness yourself! Perhaps you know the situation yourself.: dealing with a mentally ill person is not easy and it requires a lot of strength, a lot of time. Therefore, it would only make sense for you to seek professional help as well, should it be necessary. During psychotherapy, for example, you can speak openly about your fears and worries; organize your feelings and gain new perspectives.

All in all, therapy can only do you good—the same counts for self-help groups. Here you can exchange ideas with people who are also stuck or stuck in your situation. You don't have to bear the burden alone, and you will find immense understanding there. In particular, understanding is difficult to come by in everyday life, and it is simply a balm for the soul to express yourself in this way. The person you are talking to gets it honestly and sincerely. You can also benefit from the experiences within a self-help group.

Tips from other members are useful; implement them in everyday life. It is not wrong to visit a support group for relatives of people suffering from depression—more about this on our book homepage.

This is how you can tell if therapy is working

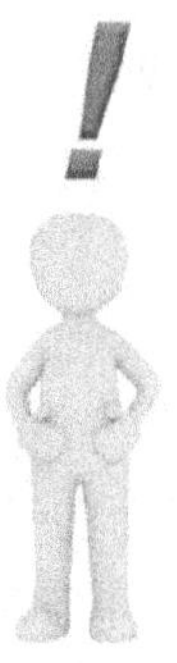

There are, of course, a myriad ways of knowing whether a therapy is working or not-- the patient's feeling is fundamental here. About 4-6 weeks after the start of therapy, drug therapy or psychotherapy, the situation should be analyzed.

This is about listening to your inner self, gladly, with the support of the practitioner. As the person concerned, if you feel that there is no progress, you should communicate this to the practitioner or therapist. If it does not fit you or the selected antidepressant does not suit you. The form of psychotherapy may also not be right for you in further experiences. Sometimes it's a combination of all three factors;

sometimes, it's just a little screw that needs to be tightened to achieve the desired success. Either way, it is important to seek open conversation and not be ashamed of it.

There is not one thing that fits everyone (be it medication, psychotherapy, or people), and just like trying on clothes, it is essential to find the right fitting over time.

You may have also noticed that you are given questionnaires at regular intervals to fill out within the therapy. These questionnaires record your current situation through specific questions. Your therapist will evaluate this and then discuss the result with you. With these questionnaires' help, tendencies can be read off whether the therapy is going in the desired direction. Getting the answers right is not an easy task with depression. After all, it may well be that you cannot distinguish the disease and its symptoms from your emotions. Here you should answer as honestly and candidly as possible. If you have any unanswered questions or feel that the therapy is not going in the desired direction, you should always seek a conversation. You can assess whether a completely new approach needs to be pursued or whether just one more step is necessary.

Consequently, the review is very important, and you should also regularly reflect or see whether the progress suits you. You are also welcome to ask family members or people around you whether they have noticed a change, no matter how small, in both a positive and a negative direction. In the end, however, it is you who decide whether the therapy should continue. All other people around you can only point out and give you tips and possibilities.

Chances of recovery

Depression is a very serious illness of the human soul. The suicide rate is high, and life with depression changes not only for those affected but also for their loved ones.

Despite all the darkness that the disease brings with it, the chances of perceiving a little more light in life are decent. The following applies: the earlier a depression is recognized, the quicker it can be treated.

If left untreated, depression is dangerous and can lead to suicide. The symptoms worsen progressively, and it can easily lead to severe depression or chronic depression. While not impossible, it is quite challenging to completely cure either of the above two forms of depression without professional help. Procrastination is similar to an infected wound: it doesn't get any better on its own. In the rarest of cases, damage limitation can only be operated! With the right drug and consistent psychotherapeutic therapy, depression can be brought under control, even cured.

Of course, some factors favor the chances of recovery:

Early detection and treatment of depression
Well adjusted antidepressants
Psychotherapy
An intact social environment
Make good use of your own resources

On the other hand, of course, there are those factors that make healing difficult:

Irregular use of antidepressants and an irregular visit to psychotherapy
Other mental illnesses, such as anxiety disorders
Inner resignation, for example, through a relapse
The environment does not accept illness, bullying
Developed addictions, for example on alcohol.

Although the chances of recovery are very good, it is still an individual point of view because the therapy of depression takes a lot of time and consistency in one's actions. It is, therefore, necessary and important to give yourself the time it takes to heal!

Statistics and Figures

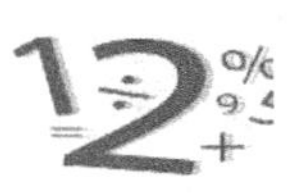 Finally, we would like to give you a few facts and figures on your way. This is often a dry topic, so we decided to put it at the end.

If you look at the global status of diseases today, cancer is in the midst of it, accounting for 8.3% of the most common diseases worldwide. Diabetes is only very rarely represented at 1.7%. 15.6% of all illnesses are at the expense of cardiovascular diseases.

Mental illnesses, including depression, account for 16.3%. The trend is increasing! Alas, it is frightening that depression is becoming increasingly common in young people. This not only means a massive personal change, but also that the good years are being lost as a result..

The tragic thing is that the population, which seems so enlightened, actually goes through life with blinkers on. Despite the knowledge of these facts and figures, it is sometimes like a fight against windmills; a grave, grave task.

A leading problem here is the maximum utilization of the health system in terms of psychotherapy. In some metropolitan areas, waiting times for outpatient psychotherapy can be a few weeks, if not months. And so, it happens that only half of those affected are treated. In some countries, it is less than 10% of the sick who receive help.

There are so many approaches and research that could save those affected from suffering or reduce it. The system load and, in some cases, overload, unfortunately also affects those involved, so that many have a longer waiting time from diagnosis to the start of psychotherapy.

Do not be discouraged by the long waiting time and use the possibilities that we have shown you here in this book, exchange ideas with others, and, if possible, get support from friends/acquaintance around you.

Author Note: In the End is the Beginning

We are now at the end of a journey through the world of depression.

What is certain is that it is possible to overcome depression and burnout and find a peaceful, mindful life full of light.
Lastly, it is time to say goodbye. But before that happens, we would like to thank you for your time, which you gave us, and this book.
We hope that you could take away some things from this book for yourself or your loved ones. If you can now understand the disease a little better, this book has already achieved a lot! It is not easy to lead a life with depression, neither for those affected nor for relatives/friends/acquaintances.

The diagnosis of burnout also means a severe blow to those affected, relatives, and work colleagues, exposed to higher stress levels. Living with such a disease is not easy, and the way back to a regulated, healthy everyday life often requires a tremendous amount of strength.

Nevertheless, the chances of recovery are very good, and it is possible to overcome depression and thus the dark side of life with one step into a more light-filled life. At first, there is a small shimmer on the horizon, which gradually becomes the rising sun. It takes time, and yet sunshine follows every rain. That's exactly how it is with depression!

But before we finally say goodbye to each other, we have one last request. If you liked this book, share it with your loved ones and help improve the mindset of the society towards depression.

If you could take a friend with you, we would be delighted to receive a recommendation and feedback. These can also be ideas, suggestions, and experiences, which we will incorporate into a future edition.

Of course, we wish you all the best for your future path, excellent health on your way out of depression! With that in mind, we would be thrilled if you read one of our other books. Until then, we would like to say goodbye to you. Do it well and stay safe!

www.ingramcontent.com/pod-product-compliance
Lightning Source LLC
Chambersburg PA
CBHW061353250726
48657CB00004B/1475